Son of Sweeney

or

Another Close Shave

A Musical Melodrama
by
Peter and Paddy Ariss

Music by Alan Breed
Lyrics by Alan Breed

CHARACTERS

Albert . . . . a barber. Known as son of Sweeney - our hero

Mrs Lovett . . . . a notorious purveyor of delectable pies

A Stranger . . . . whose identity *will be revealed*

Jonah Grubb . . . . a barber's assistant

Tobias Wragg . . . . his friend and colleague

Captain Nelson Thumbtickle . . . . a seafaring type

Miss Emily Raven . . . . an emancipated woman
a journalist and our heroine

P.C. Fred Birkentwit . . . . the pride of Scotland Yard

P.C. Bill Wally . . . . another of the same

Faith, Hope and Charity . . . . Ladies of the night
(no better than they should be)

Maisie, Bess and Liz   chorus of Pie Makers, all sweet and tasty

A Man in Black . . . . another stranger

Customers, street vendors, street urchins, passers-by, peelers, pick-pockets, etc.

ACT I

The year is 1888, or thereabouts, and the place is Fleet Street, London. Much of the action takes place on the front portion of the stage, which represents the street itself; towards the back of the stage is a row of shops, the central one being a Barber's Shop, complete with striped pole. (If the stage is large, the Bakery may also be seen stage left of the barber's but in darkness). Across the open frontage of the shop there are three chairs, and behind them is a table with jugs, basins, towels, scissors, and so on. There is a doorway at the rear of the shop, and on the left can be seen part of the next-door Pie Shop. There are exits DL and DR from the street. When the curtain rises, the shop stays in shadow as the front of the stage gradually comes up to full 'daylight'.

The scene opens with 28 bars of Orchestra which reflects the Bells of

London. The following NINE Street Cries, which make up the prologue to the Son of Sweeney, are interchangeable and/or removable. The harmonic structure is such that any one Street Cry can replace any other, provided entry is made at the right place in the 4 Bar pattern. Furthermore, the Street Cries can be reduced to ONE ONLY (repeated incessantly or occasionally) if the cast is small, or, alternatively, new Street Cries can be created and added ad infinitum - and the 4 Bar pattern extended if a large cast is to be accommodated.

The nine Street Cries, in the order in which they occur on the manuscript, are:-

1. Oh, what a great morning for singing;
Sure is a great morning for shaking off the blues.

2. Who will buy my sweet-scented lavender?
Only tuppence a large colourful spray.

3. I'll sharpen up your razors, your rusty knives I'll grind.
I'm recognized (b'Jaysus) as the best you'll ever find.

4. Pies, succulent pies; juicy meat pies,
A feast for your eyes.

5. Eels, alive-o, eels alive-o! Jellied or roasted
Or sauteed or stewed.

6. Matches for sale, matches for sale.
Each of my lucifers lights without fail.

7. If you've any broken chairs to mend,
Then to you my skills I do extend.

8. Bright yellow daffodils, sprinkled with dew;
Snowdrops and crocuses, 'specially for you.

9. "Oranges and Lemons" say the bells of St. Clements,
"You owe me five farthings", say the bells of St.Martins.

(While the singers are in full flow, a cockney woman lets out a piercing scream - see music. Her male partner asks:)

MAN: What's the matter?

WOMAN: Isn't that the very shop where the Demon Barber of Fleet Street slaughtered his many victims?

MAN: D'you mean Sweeney Todd?

2nd MAN: He was odd!

3rd MAN: Sweeney Todd?

4th MAN: Oh my God!

OPENING CHORUS

MEN: Sweeney Todd was a barber with the sharpest intellect,

WOMEN: Sweeney Todd was a barber and an architect.

MEN: Sweeney Todd was a barber who'd inspect and select or reject everyone that he shaved.

WOMEN: Sweeney Todd was a barber with a cutting repartee.

MEN: Sweeney Todd was a barber and a rarity;

WOMEN: Sweeney Todd was a barber, full of glee, who'd agree to relieve you of all that you'd saved.

ALL: Just the strong and the brave would ask him for a shave.

MEN: Sweeney Todd was a barber with a gushing clientele,

WOMEN: Sweeney Todd was a barber with a tale to tell.

MEN: Sweeney Todd was a barber who'd propel you pell-mell off to hell with a yell and a wave.

WOMEN: All is well now he's gone to the grave.

ALL: We're saved!

(At the end of the number the chorus exeunt, leaving only the three barbers, two customers, the CAPTAIN, EMILY writing in her notebook DR, and the STRANGER DL. As the last member of the chorus exits, and the CAPTAIN heads for the centre chair in the barber's shop, the voice of a Town Crier is heard calling)

CRIER: All's well in London Town! Eight of the clock, and all's well!

(The lights fade, and a green spot shines on the STRANGER.)

STRANGER: *(aside)* All's well? Hah! Ha ha ha ha! He he he ! All's well!!

(With a final burst of maniacal laughter, the STRANGER exits DR. The lights come up, focusing on the barber's shop.)

ALBERT: Good morning, Sir! What will it be? A shave? Or a short back and sides, sir?

CAPTAIN: No, no, just a trim, thank you. *(General 'rhubarb' as all the customers are attended to by the three barbers.)* Who was the mysterious gentleman in the black cloak and top hat? He seemed very... I don't know... well mysterious!

ALBERT: I've seen him once or twice lately, and he reminds me of someone but I can't think who it could be. Anyway, it's difficult to tell, with his face all muffled up like that. Do you know who he is, Jonah?

JONAH: *(busy with his customer)* Nah.

TOBIAS: Me neither. But I don't much like the looks of him, smart though he may be.

ALBERT: Someone told me he'd just come back from abroad.

CAPTAIN: There's a coincidence - so have I.

ALBERT: Really, sir? A seafaring gentleman, I take it?

CAPTAIN: That's right, my boy. And who'd have thought it? Nearly twenty years ago I was press -ganged -

JONAH: Walking along Fleet Street, was you?

CAPTAIN: *(Surprised)* Yes, I was! I was pres-ganged, forced to go to sea and abandon my wife and the child she was soon to bear; yet now I have my own ship, and have sailed the seven seas in her. Captain Nelson Thumbtickle is the name.

ALBERT: Proud to make your acquaintance, Captain. It's good to see a man who's overcome adversity and prospered. You hear that, Jonah?

JONAH: *(Still busy)* Nah.

TOBIAS: I heard. Glad to meet you, sir. *(He leans over, shakes hands, then gets back to work).*

ALBERT: What brings you to London, Captain?

CAPTAIN: My ship' being victualled for her next voyage, and meanwhile I have some business here - unfinished business from nearly twenty years ago. *(Pause)* Who is this Sweeney Todd they were all talking about just now? *(ALBERT looks embarrassed and turns away. TOBIAS cuts in.)*

TOBIAS: Sweeney Todd was his father, Captain. Used to own this very shop, sir, a barber he was, but about ten years back he took to robbing and murdering his customers, and made 'em into pies with the help of his accomplice Mrs. Lovett, her what had the pie shop next door.

CAPTAIN: *(Aside)* Mrs. Lovett! Can it be? No, surely not... although *my* Mrs. Lovett did make excellent pies... *(To TOBIAS, casually)* What happened to them?

TOBIAS: Sweeney was condemned to be hanged...

JONAH: He got a suspended sentence...

TOBIAS: - and Mrs. Lovett was sent to prison for life, when she recovered from Sweeney's murderous attack upon her. They both went to Newgate Gaol, and Mrs. Lovett worked in the kitchens -

JONAH: She was doing porridge...

TOBIAS: - as she was famous for her cooking. She helped Sweeney escape - the hangman had an off-day and tied a granny knot -

JONAH: No noose is good news!

TOBIAS: *-and* the rope broke, and Mrs. L. Managed to smuggle Sweeney out in a rubbish cart...

JONAH: Best place for him, with the rubbish.

TOBIAS: - and he escaped, abroad we think. Anyway, nobody's seen him for ten years or so.

CAPTAIN: Mmmm... and what of - Mrs. Lovett?

ALBERT: They released her from gaol.

TOBIAS: Oh yes, Albert, so they did. But let's tell the Captain *why* they released her, eh? Mrs. Lovett is Albert's mother, sir, so he don't like to speak no ill of her, you understand. As it happens, she's not a bad sort really, and she got worried 'cos all the prisoners was all so thin and that, so she started improving their victuals by adding meat; the only way she could get meat was to chop up any prisoners wot died, and she made them into pies. Very nutritious they was, I'm told, and the prisoners got 'ealthier, and then they started to hurry things along a bit in order to find the ingredients for the pies.

JONAH: More went into gaol than ever came out.

TOBIAS: The Governor got suspicious after a while, and when the chief warder went missing...

JONAH: - *and* the prison cat...

TOBIAS: - he decided enough was enough and expelled Mrs. L. from the prison. She came back to Albert, and her pie shop.

ALBERT: Without Sweeney's evil influence and his blackmail she has worked hard and made a *good* reputation with her pies and pastries.

JONAH: He means they don't have anything in them wot they shouldn't.

CAPTAIN: *(carefully)* And where is this pie shop?

ALBERT: *(Pointing L.)* Right next door.

CAPTAIN: Really! Well, I'd better be off.

EMILY: *(Scribbling)* I didn't get that?

CAPTAIN: Be off.

EMILY: *(slightly shocked)* Oh!

CAPTAIN: Thank you. Albert, is it? Here's sixpence - keep the change.

ALBERT: *(Impressed)* Thank you very much, sir.

CAPTAIN: And you're Mrs. Lovett's boy... how old are you, Albert?

ALBERT: Nearly twenty, sir.

CAPTAIN: *(staring at ALBERT)* Hmmm... it could be... what happened to you while Mrs. Lovett was - um - away?

ALBERT: I was taken in and cared for by Mrs. Raven, who lives across the street there, next to the shoemakers.

EMILY: I missed that?

JONAH: Cobblers.

EMILY: Oh.

JONAH: He's sweet on Mrs. Raven's daughter Emily.

TOBIAS: That's her over there - she's a reporter.

ALBERT: Nonsense, Jonah - we're like brother and sister, that's all. We were brought up together.

TOBIAS: When Albert got old enough, he opened up the shop again and give me my old job back, only more like a partner, see.

CAPTAIN: I see. Very interesting indeed. Hmmm. *(For a moment he stands deep in thought, then turns abruptly and exits DL.)*

TOBIAS: Well! Bit of a nosy parker, weren't he?

ALBERT: *(Bitterly)* Just natural curiosity, I expect - I find people always want to dig up all that old scandal about my mother and father. My father deserves it, damn him, but my mother would never have done anything wrong if he hadn't forced her into it.

TOBIAS: Maybe so, maybe not.

JONAH: What's it matter, anyway?

ALBERT: *(hotly)* It matters to *me.*

TOBIAS: Aw, c'mon, lets forget it. Why don't we cheer ourselves up? Let's do our Barber Shop Quartet.

JONAH: How can it be a Quartet when there's only three of us?

TOBIAS: *(simply)* Why not?

ALBERT: Good question! Let's go...

(The Three Barbers sing:-)

SWEET CAROLINE

Oh Caroline, sweet Caroline,
Your arms entwine with mine, with mine;
Like sparkling wine, your eyes divine
Will ever shine in mine, in mine.

Oh Caroline, sweet Caroline,
Your thoughts align with mine, with mine.
Just give a sign, your heart resign

And say you're mine, all mine.
Just say you're mine!

(At the conclusion of the song, the customers applaud, pay their bills to the barbers, then make their exits amidst general 'rhubarb' - "Good night!" "Thank you, sir", "Watch out for the ripper!" "Ha ha!" etc. EMILY now comes forward, as TOBIAS and JONAH bust themselves tidying the shop, and later confer quietly together at the back of the shop. Lights fade slightly on the shop, as ALBERT steps forward into the street.)

ALBERT: Emily! I haven't seen you for days - where *have* you been?

EMILY: *(Mysteriously)* Oh - around. Just around.

ALBERT: I do hope you're not still on the trail of the Ripper. You could get yourself killed.

EMILY: *(Coyly)* Would you miss me?

ALBERT: Of course I would! We all would! Emily, please will you promise me that you won't do anything silly?

EMILY: Oh dear. You *know* how difficult it is for me - nobody takes me seriously because I'm a girl, and I have to work twice as hard to prove I can be just a s good as any of the other reporters.

ALBERT: The Whitechapel Gazette is hardly a suitable paper for a young lady to work for.

EMILY: There you go! You're as bad as the rest. The Gazette is perfectly suitable for me, thank you, and I intend to make a success of it if it's the last thing I do.

ALBERT: That's what I'm afraid of - that it *will* be the last thing you do. The Ripper *kills*. Emily - kills brutally and horribly. How can I describe it to you - you, with your delicate sensibilities?

EMILY: *(Calmly)* Delicate sensibilities, my foot. I know exactly what the Ripper does to his victims - I saw one of them last week, just before the peelers arrived on the scene. It's very nasty, I admit, but then that's all the more reason to find out who the Ripper is, and catch him before he murders all the girls in Whitechapel.

ALBERT: Emily - you're wonderful. You really are! But why can't you leave it to the police? They're properly trained to handle murderers.

EMILY: Don't worry, I shall keep out of his way - P.C. Wally and his men can do all the handling when the time comes. But first *someone* has to find out who he really is - there are so many wild rumours hurtling around just now. I even heard one suggesting that he may be a member of the Royal Family! Imagine! What would our dear Queen think?... Now, I have a theory, and I'm pretty certain I'm right, too, but - *(she stops suddenly.)*

ALBERT: Well? What is it/ What were you going to say?

EMILY: *(lamely)* Er, well, no. I can't say anything yet.

ALBERT: Why? Not even to me?

EMILY: *(Softly)* Especially not to you.

ALBERT: I don't understand. *(He turns away upstage, towards the shop.)*

EMILY: *(sadly)* You will, my dear, you will. *(Then, aside)* I love him! How can I tell him that I suspect Jack the Ripper to be none other than his own father?

(EMILY sings "The Boy I Love".)

> The boy I love eclipses ev'ry star,
> His sparkling eyes have brightened up the sky,
> The boy I love I keep dreaming of,
> And the magic of my dreams will never die.
>
> The boy I love is quite the best by far,
> His winning smile has captured ev'ry eye;
> The boy I love I keep dreaming of,
> And I know my love for him will never die.
>
> In his loving arms I long to be,
> How I yearn for hie caress!
> Could his lonely heart belong to me?
> Could I know true happiness?
>
> The boy I love knows what my feelings are,
> His tender words could banish ev'ry sigh;
> The boy I love I keep dreaming of,
> But I guess he'll stay a dream until I die.
>
> In his loving arms I long to be,

How I yearn for his caress!
Could his lonely heart belong to me?
Could I know true happiness?

The boy I love knows what my feelings are,
And yet he fails to hear my plaintive cry;
The boy I love I keep dreaming of,
For I know I could provide him,
With the love that's been denied him;
He must need me there beside him, or I'll die.

(EMILY exits DL. ALBERT looks sadly after her, as the lights fade to denote the passage of time. This may be emphasised by either a programme note, or by the way of a sign carried by a street urchin. It is now late the same evening. The scene is exactly as before.)

ALBERT: All right, Tobias, Jonah - you can get off home now. I don't think we're likely to get any more customers in tonight.

TOBIAS: I'll lock up, if you like. I'm not in any hurry.

JONAH: I am - got a girl waiting for me. Good night! *(He rushes off, DL, pulling on his jacket.)*

ALBERT: Thanks, Tobias.

TOBIAS: Are you all right, Albert? You seem a bit down.

ALBERT: Yes, of course I'm all right. No I'm not. I'm just worried about Emily.

TOBIAS: Why don't you marry the girl and have done with it? Then you could keep a proper eye on her. Land her with a bunch of kids, and she'll have no time for all this gallivanting.

ALBERT: Oh, Toby, if only I could!

TOBIAS: What's stopping you, for heaven's sake? She loves you too, don't she?

ALBERT: I think so - but how *can* I? A pure, sensitive, lovely, virtuous, innocent maiden like Emily - what have I to offer her but the tainted blood of a murderer? My father, Sweeney Todd!

TOBIAS: I see your point. But I reckon Miss Emily is much too sensible to worry over a little thing like that.

ALBERT: *(Wallowing in self pity)* I can never wed. Never!

TOBIAS: Suit yourself.

ALBERT: *(After a pause)* She's so brave, so wonderfully brave, but - the Ripper!

TOBIAS: He's only killed street girls so far. As far as we know that is. Maybe he wouldn't go for a young lady like her.

ALBERT: If he finds out she's on to him, there's no knowing what he'll do.

TOBIAS: If any girl can take care of herself, it's Miss Emily. Now off you go - see if you can find her.

(Exit ALBERT DL. TOBIAS sighs, shrugs, picks up a copy of the Whitechapel Gazette, swivels round in one of the chairs until his back is to the audience, and starts to read. Enter SWEENEY,

Green Spot, as all the other lights dim. The ensuing speech should be accompanied by occasional dramatic chords on the piano.)

SWEENEY: *(Aside)* Aha! Ha ha ha! These fools are all wondering who I am, wondering who is the mysterious stranger in their midst! Little do they know that it is I, Sweeney Todd, the Demon Barber of Fleet street, returning to the scene of the nefarious crimes! *(He flings back his cloak.)* I, with the mark of the rope around me neck! The scar of the hangman's noose! *(He pulls down his muffler to show a bright red mark on his neck.)* The mark of Cain... When I first escaped I went overseas - to the Isle of Wight. Then for ten long years I terrorised the far countries of the world, but now, with the police forces of every continent hot upon me trail, I have come back to me old haunts, the one place where nobody would ever expect to find me! And I have found a new source of satisfaction for me surgical talents - carving up street girls! Pah! No-one will miss them. People are calling me Jack the Ripper! The fools. Ha ha ha! So far I have foiled them all. But - there is one little problem. Disposing of the bodies. The best brains of Scotland Yard are pitted against me - yet they have found only five of the twenty seven disembowelled bodies upon which it has been my pleasure to operate.

However! I have just heard that me old friend and partner Mrs. Lovett is not as dead as I thought she was when I slit her throat ten years ago, and is in fact back in business at her pie shop. I knew, of course, that she had survived me murderous attack upon her, for the foolish woman even helped me to escape from prison - and the hangman. Indeed, I am so grateful that I feel I really must call upon her, and thank her for her kindness to me all those years ago! Ha! And where better to dispose of me surplus sweetmeats than in her tasty pies? I shall pay a visit to my dear Mrs. L., and *persuade* her to join me in a lucrative little venture once again. She never could resist me charms or me threats. But wait! Curses! Someone comes. *(He retreats into the shadows, UR. The lights are raised front of stage as three Street Girls enter, two DL and one DR, nervously looking over their shoulders. One of the Customers enters, also P.C. WALLY and P.C. BIRKENTWIT, and a street vendor or two. The opening music plays softly in the background. The girls try to keep their minds on the job by picking up some men, but their hearts are not in it and they have no luck. They end up together centre stage, the others exiting at opposite points to their respective entrances. FAITH, HOPE, and CHARITY sing their first part of the song.)*

We were six tarts when we started,
Now we're three who're broken hearted,
'Cos the half of us have been done in,
We're not feeling very chirper
'Cos we think it's Jack the Ripper,
So we're comforting ourselves with gin.
It's the duty of the strumpet
To supply men with some crumpet,
And to give 'em all an easy lay,
It's our privilege as trollops
To provide raw sex in dollops,
And no matter what the time of day
Our professional belief is to give a man relief,
For relief is what the game is all about,
If the meeting's only brief,
Then they think we're like a thief,
'Cos a thief takes all he can, without a doubt,
It's a pleasure for the scrubber,

Dressed in leather, silk or ribber,
Or in calico or pink chiffon,
So to titillate the clients.
With techniques unknown to science
That she'll satisfy the paying john
With whatever seems to turn him on.

FAITH: Oh well, back to work, I suppose. I'm just *so* tired, I've been up and down them stairs to my room all day.

HOPE: Oh, your poor *feet.*

FAITH: How's business with you then, dear?

HOPE: Got a weird one yesterday. Up from the country somewhere - Gloucester, I think he said. It figured.

CHARITY: What d'you mean, it figured?

HOPE: Well, he was like the Seven Bore - the type that only comes up once a year. *(The girls shriek with laughter.)*

CHARITY: Almost as good as mine - he couldn't tell incest from arson. Set his sister on fire, he told me. *(More laughter.)*

FAITH: Mmm...One of mine reminded me of what my mother used to tell me - lie back and think of England. *He* reminded me of *Wilts*hire. Or maybe *Middle*sex...

HOPE: They say this Jack the Ripper might be Royalty. You ever 'ad Royalty?

CHARITY: No, not me, but me grandma did. Said he used to fondle her orbs while she played with his spectre.

HOPE: Oh, go *on*, you're a scream, you are! *(Laughter.)*

FAITH: ...or Nor*thampton*...

HOPE: Wot *are* you going on about?

FAITH: *(Still miles away)*...Or *Little*hampton - yes, that was more like it.

CHARITY: Ooh, look, here comes the peelers.

HOPE: They can't be after us - there's not a toff in sight. *(Enter P.C.WALLY and BIRKENTWIT.)* We ain't done nothing. Give us a break.

BILL: That's all right, girls, you can relax.

FRED: *We* ain't after you, not today we ain't - but Jack the Ripper might be, so you'd better be very careful who you talk to.

CHARITY: Thanks for the warning, but we had heard.

FAITH: Not 'arf. Ugh.

HOPE: Fair gives us the shivers, it does.

BILL: We'll get him, girls, don't you fret.

FAITH: Sure you will. But how many more of our mates is he going to do in first? There's more wot 'as disappeared than 'as ever been found, you know.

HOPE: Remember that girl from Glasgow? The one we couldn't understand a word she was saying?

CHARITY: Nor she couldn't understand us, neither - yeah, I remember. That's wot Did for her, I reckon - didn't know wot we was talking about when we warned her to watch out.

BILL: *(Obviously smitten by her charms)* Your name's Charity, ain't it?

CHARITY: Don't get smart ideas - I don't give nothing away for free. And I know wot you're going to say - how come I'm called Charity when the fellers have to pay for it? Well, my ma nearly called me Virginia, but that don't make no sense either, do it?

FAITH: Funny thing about names. I went to church once, and the preacher kept saying "'Ave Faith! 'Ave Faith!" And he did too. Fourteen times.

FRED: *(Laughing)* That's a good 'un! How about you, Hope?

HOPE: *(Sexily)* I'm Hope because I'm abandoned, and pleasure all who enter here...*(Laughter. Girls sing again.)*

FAITH: I'm Faith -

HOPE: I'm Hope -

CHARITY: I'm Charity -

GIRLS: And we all love familiarity -
          We would proposition slave or king;
          But we'd like to drown our troubles

In a sea of champagne bubbles
And forget about the whole damn thing,
In a world as bad as this is,
Where true ignorance is bliss,
We can teach our men the lesson's they require;
They can call me "Hit and Miss",
Stand upon the precipice,
Even give my arms a kiss if they desire.

CHARITY: *(With a sudden shiver)* I don't know why we're all standing here laughing. The Ripper ain't funny.

FAITH: Anyway, we got to get back to work - I'm broke. My gentleman friend touched me for a quid last night.

HOPE: Cor, you've upped yer prices, ain't yer, darling?

FAITH: Oh, you! *(She hits her playfully.)*

CHARITY: Come on you two, that's enough.

FRED: Don't even go with the toffs you've been with before.

HOPE: It's hard enough to earn a living as it is - if we want to eat, we go with the fellers.

FRED: It's just a friendly warning. Don't go with men.

BILL: Unless it's us!

FAITH: That'll be the day. When we give it to a hard up peeler.

BILL: No joking, girls. Like he said - watch it. Now get along home - and remember: *Be Careful.*

FAITH: Ta.

HOPE: Come on, girls.

CHARITY: Ta-ra, then.

BILL: Ta-ra, girls.

FRED: Ta-ra.

(Exeunt the girls DR and the policemen DL. CHARITY gives a come-on to BILL as she goes: he turns to follow her, but FRED steers him firmly in the

opposite direction. SWEENEY now steps forward again. Green spotlight.)

SWEENEY: Ha! At last, they've gone! So! Now to approach Mrs. L. and prevail upon her to join me in me evil plans. But what is this? Curses! I am foiled, yet again! I must bide me time...

(He shrinks back into the shadows, listening, as MRS. LOVETT enters UL and goes over to TOBIAS. The lights come up on the shop.)

MRS L: *(Calling)* Tobias! Tobias! Oh there you are. You *are* working late tonight.

SWEENEY: *(aside)* It is she!

TOBIAS: Just clearing up for Albert so that he can go chasing off after Miss Emily.

MRS L: Ah me! Young love, young love...

TOBIAS: Mrs Lovett, there's something I've been meaning to ask you.

MRS L: Yes, Tobias?

TOBIAS: Well, I hope you don't mind me asking, but I was only about ten when all the trouble happened here - I was just an apprentice barber to that evil monster Sweeney Todd, and saved from his murderous knife by the timely intervention of Eelpie the Gypsy.

SWEENEY: *(Aside)* Curses! The brat Tobias!

MRS L: Get on with it, lad.

TOBIAS: I don't remember much about it - it was all so very confusing, and I had only just started to work here that very day. But I got the impression that the pie shop lady was done in - and I'm sure she was called Mrs. Lovett too. *Was* it you?

MRS L: *(Sighing)* Yes, Tobias, it was. Sweeney thought he'd killed me - he slit my throat, the swine - but the prison doctors were able to save me.

TOBIAS: So that's it. I thought I must be right.

SWEENEY: *(Aside)* This boy is dangerous! What if he recognises me too, and denounces me to the officers of the Law? He cannot be allowed to live. *He must die!*

MRS L: I came back here for Albert's sake. He was only a lad at the time too, about your own age near enough, and as luck would have it was away working for old Mistress Parkin in Pudding Lane at the time of the final bloody episode, so he knew nothing about it till he got home. Mrs Raven kindly took him in - me already having been took off to prison - and she bought him up along with Emily while I was away. It was a bad time for him, knowing his ma was in gaol and believing his father to be a murderer.

TOBIAS: He's still worrying about that - says he can't ask Miss Emily to marry him because the blood of Sweeney Todd runs in his veins.

SWEENEY: *(stepping forward and throwing back his cloak)* Did anyone call?

MRS L: *(In horror)* Sweeney? Can it be. Oh, no! No, no, no! It cannot be! Yes, it can. Is it? It is! Sweeney Todd!

SWEENEY: I can see you are quite overcome with emotion at this happy reunion, me dear Mrs. L . But me erstwhile apprentice knows too much, methinks. And I know only one sure way to be sure he keeps silent - as silent as the grave.

MRS L: *No*, Mr. T.! No, no! *Please* don't start that all over again!

SWEENEY: Start again, me dear? I have never stopped!

TOBIAS: Touch me if you dare! I am not a puny ten-year-old now! I'm going for the Law!

(He turns to go.)

SWEENEY: Oh no you're not. *(He grabs him as he passes, and TOBIAS puts up a brave struggle.)*Die! *(He plunges a dagger into TOBIAS'S chest.)* Die! *(And again.)* Die! *(And again)* Ha ha ha! He he he!

(TOBIAS enjoys his death scene, MRS.L. is sobbing with her hands over her face, powerless to help, and the curtain falls to the sound of SWEENEY's maniacal laughter.)

END OF ACT I

ACT II

(Three days have passed. The action takes place in the bakery below the pie shop - as before, this is set towards the back of the stage, open-fronted, with

Fleet Street in the foreground. The lighting indicates where the scene is taking place; in the bakery or on the street.

There are two trestle tables centre stage, on which are rolling pins, flour, basins, etc. Along the back wall are ovens. There is a door DL leading upstairs to the shop, and a door UL to the laundry room. A concealed door lies centre R. Just downstage of this stands a large hamper, with a huge padlock on it. Big earthenware jars marked flour, sugar, salt etc stand by the tables. The three pie makers - MAISIE, BESSIE and LIZZIE - are busy, each with a rolling pin, as they sing the first part of their song. They get a bit carried away and start flicking flour and pies at each other. Song; "Luvverly Pies".)

> Luvverly pies! Luvverly Pies!
> Lovett's pies are juicy and fine.
> Just oozing with gravy and heady as wine,
> Full of young lamb or fresh chicken or veal -
> Only one pie makes an excellent meal
> Excellent meal! Oodles of veal!
> Lovett's pies are flavoured so well
> With spices and tasty herbs; that's why they sell,
> That's why they're selling so terribly well.
> Crusty pies, tender and sweet,
> Lovett's pies are a luvverly treat!
> Luvverly pies are still in their prime,
> We're busy as bees, about all of the time;
> Luvverly pies, and oh, what a good meal -
> Full of thick gravy, prime pork and fresh veal .
> Luvverly pies...luvverly pies...

MAISIE: Oh, stop it Bessie, do - Mrs. L. won't half give you what-for if she comes down from the shop!

BESSIE: She'll give us *all* what-for)giggling) But it's more fun than baking pies! *(She hurls a pie at LIZZIE.)*

LIZZIE: Oooh, just look at the mess! *(She hurls a pie too.)*

BESSIE: Mind you - ouch! That *hurt*! - Mrs. L. Can hardly give us the sack, can she?

MAISIE: Why ever not?

BESSIE: Well, there's been funny goings-on the last few days - don't say you haven't noticed.

MAISIE: You mean - that big hamper? With the padlock 'n all?

LIZZIE: And Mrs. L. Crying all over the place, and hiding in the laundry room half the time?

BESSIE: It's a rum do, ain't it. I can't make it out.

LIZZIE: Nor, me.

BESSIE: Me neither. Anyway, whatever it is, she won't want us telling nobody, now will she? Not after the trouble she had last time. Oh me gawd - someone's coming! Quick - get busy girls.*(They rush forward, but soon relax again as P.C.BILL WALLY and P.C. FRED BIRKENTWIT enter DL, from the shop)* Oh, it's only Bill and Fred! That's a relief. Still, we'd better be'ave ourselves now the Law's 'ere.

BESSIE: That'll be the day! What do you want, boys! Sweet or savoury?

BILL: I'll have a jammy one, please. Never been too certain of the meat pies, not since Mrs.L. had her little spot of bother a few years back.

MAISIE: Ten years, for heaven's sake!

LIZZIE: And they really are scrumptious - everybody says so.

BESSIE: You *know* she don't get up to nothing like that now. *(Virtuously)* We could never consider working here if she did.

BILL: Garn - you know I'm only teasing.

FRED: I always prefer a tasty tart, meself *(Leering at the girls)* but I'll have a meat pie today, just to show willing.

MAISIE: *(Dishing out the pies)* It's a wonder we ever makes any profit here, all the pies we gives away.

BILL: *(Leering playfully)* You just can't resist us handsome fellows, that's wot it is. And wot's more, we're willing too!

MAISIE: *(Sharply)* Ah, but are you able?

FRED: Looks like this pie's been crimped with a set of false teeth.

LIZZIE: Just be thankful we're not making doughnuts today - you'd be surprised wot we makes the holes with sometimes.

MAISIE: Look, give us a hand, will you, if you can spare a minute - we got to clear up this mess before Mrs. L. comes in and catches us. Here, Freddy - catch! *(She hurls a pie at him - and in a moment all 5 of them are involved in another messy battle.)*

FRED: Cripes - look at ne uniform! I can't go on the street looking like this!

LIZZIE: *(Sexily)* Come into the laundry room with me - I'll give you a rub-down...*(They exit UL.)*

BILL: Well, that's a bit of all right - come on, Maisie, give us a hand with my uniform, will you?

MAISIE: Never miss an opportunity, do you? *(They move UL.)*

BESSIE: Don't be long, you girls, I'm not cleaning all this up on me own.

MAISIE: Why not - you're a scrubber, ain't yer?

(She ducks as BESSIE throws a pie at her, and she and BILL exit UL.)

BESSIE: Oh lord, Mrs. L.'s sure to be down to collect fresh pies and cakes for the shop. Oh! The cakes! They must be ready! *(She rushes to the ovens and takes out a tray or two of cakes. Humming to herself, she puts them on the table, and places a tray of pies in the oven. She starts cleaning up, until BILL and FRED enter with LIZZIE and MAISIE, UL.)*

BILL: That's a bit better - wouldn't do to get into trouble with the Sergeant, would it, Fred?

FRED: Right. *(Takes another pie and starts eating.)*

MAISIE: It's a wonder you two aren't as fat as elephants, the way you scoffs our pies every day.

BILL: Be fair, Maisie. It ain't *every* day.

FRED: We're not on duty *every* day!

BILL: And anyway - we does our little bit to keep fit, don't we, Fred?

FRED: Let's show them.

(Song "Keep fit". Girls watch in admiration.)

BILL:	I must do m'little bit to keep fit; I must do m'little bit to keep fit; Mother nature had a plan - 'Twas to make of me a man. I must do m'little bit to keep fit.
FRED:	I must do m'little bit to keep fit; I must do m'little bit to keep fit; Ev'ry crook'll weep and wail As I wheel 'em off to jail, If I do m'little bit to keep fit.

BILL: This is it, m'little bit to keep fit.

FRED: That was it? Your little bit to keep fit?

BILL: I have done m'little bit to keep fit.

FRED: Overdone 'is little bit to keep fit.

BILL: I'm the pick of every force -

FRED: In good nick as well, of course!

BOTH: That was it - our little bit to keep fit.

BILL: Oh, sh...ugar!

(The song should be accompanied by actions - the odd knees-bend and so on, requiring little exertion but apparently causing considerable back-ache. As the song ends, MRS. LOVETT enters.)

MRS L: *(Standing still as she surveys the chaos)* Well! And just what do you girls think you're doing? And you two *(She points at the men)* - you ought to know better than to encourage them. Go on - off you go. *(BILL and FRED exit DL, rather shamefacedly, grabbing an extra cake or two on their way.)*

MAISIE: Sorry, Mrs. Lovett. We was just having a bit of fun.

MRS L: Fun? Fun! On *my* time? Oh, this is the last straw. *Look* at all this mess - and customers waiting upstairs for their fresh pies. *(She starts to cry.)*

BESSIE: *(Contritely)* We didn't mean no harm, honest. Look, there's a bun in the oven - Lizzie! Don't say it, I know you! - and there's some cakes ready and waiting, I'll take them up now. *(She takes trays of cakes and exits* *quickly DL.)*

LIZZIE: Don't cry, Mrs. Lovett - we'll clear it all up, really we will. *(The girls get busy)*

MRS L: *(stifling her sobs)* Maisie - fetch the cloths and things from the laundry room.

MAISIE: Yes, Mrs. Lovett. *(She does so. BESS returns, DL and the 3 girls, humming their tune, clear up. MRS. L. has moved R, and is staring at the hamper.)* What *is* in that big basket, Mrs Lovett? All locked up like that, it can't be just laundry, surely.

MRS L: Don't ask, child, don't ask. I dread to think... it reminds me of ... no, it can't be.

MAISIE: Mr. Brown bought it and said we wasn't to touch it.

MRS L: Mr. Brown?

MAISIE: Yes - that tall bloke with the black cloak and the big muffler.

MRS L: Oh yes. Mr. Brown. Yes...

MAISIE: He's a stranger in these parts, ain't he?

MRS L: *Very* strange - but no stranger.

MAISIE: Huh? I haven't seen him before - well, not before he started work at the barber's shop a couple of days ago.

MRS L: It was before your time, Maisie. Nearly ten years now.

LIZZIE: It seems odd that a gent like him should be *working.*

BESSIE: *(sharply)* That's quite enough of your gossiping. Those pies should be ready by now - take them upstairs, you can all go and mind the shop for a bit while I finish tidying up in here. Perhaps you won't get into so much trouble up there.

GIRLS: Thank you, Mrs Lovett. *(They exit DL, giggling, one carrying a tray of pies which she has taken from the oven. MRS LOVETT goes over to the concealed door R, and opens it. SWEENEY is standing in the opening with the green spotlight on him. She shrieks and drops the metal bucket she is carrying.)*

MRS L: *You!*

SWEENEY: *(looking back over his shoulder)* Who?

MRS L: Vile murderer!

SWEENEY: *(modestly)* True...

MRS L: What do you want? Is it not enough that I went to gaol for you? Is it not enough that I bribed the hangman and helped you escape the gallows - a fate you so richly deserved? Why must you haunt me like this - haunt me, and taunt me, and hound me? Can I never be free of you?

SWEENEY: *Dear* Mrs. L. Do take care. You are likely to burst a blood-vessel if you continue in this vein.

MRS L: Murderer! Torturer! Damned villain!!!

SWEENEY: Come, come, me dear. Your histrionics are beginning to bore me. You and I have much to talk about -

MRS L: I never, ever, want to talk to you again.

SWEENEY: -and I rather think you have been trying to avoid me, ever since that unfortunate little contretemps with Master Tobias. So sad - to die so young.

MRS L: *(momentarily diverted)* Contra - what?

SWEENEY: Contretemps. A useful french phrase which I picked up - amongst other things! - upon me travels across the five continents.

MRS L: Oh. Well - I still have nothing to say to you - not now, not ever. And particularly after what you did to poor Toby, who never did you any harm to anybody. How *could* you?

SWEENEY: *(grinning fiendishly)* Very easily, me dear, as you saw for yourself. However, even if you have nothing to say to me, I have a considerable amount to say to *you*, me dear old friend and partner in crime.

MRS L: Not so much of the partner, if you please! All over and done with, that is, and paid for with three years in gaol - though *you* got away scot-free, *which*, I may remind you, was all thanks to *me*, and if you have any gratitude in that black heart of yours you will show it by leaving me alone.

SWEENEY: You are remarkably loquacious, madam, for one who has sworn never to speak to me again. Well, well, well! Gratitude? Hah! Now *that* is a word I did *not* pick up on me travels. I do not know the meaning of the word. Surely you did not expect gratitude from Sweeney Todd?

You, who know me so well? You amaze me! *(He grabs her by the wrist.)* Enough of this. To business. You will work for me again, as you did before.

MRS L: No! No! No! No, I will *not*! I know you have taken Toby's place in the shop next door - shame on you! - but your fiendish barber's chair was dismantled years ago; there is no longer any way in which you can tip your victims down into the cellar from above, as you used to do.

SWEENEY: A trifling inconvenience, dear lady. Will it surprise you to learn that I now have *other* sources of supply? Admittedly there is little in the way of gold and jewels to be had there, but the flesh is even more tender, and I have a yearning - yes, a *yearning*, Mrs. Lovett, to savour one of your delicious pies again.

MRS L: No, no a thousand times no! I will not. I refuse. I would rather die!

SWEENEY: *(suavely)* That can be arranged.

MRS L: *(Sobbing)* I hate you. I despise you.

SWEENEY: Tut.

MRS L: *(In a low clear voice)* I - will - not - cook - for - you.

SWEENEY: *(Amused)* Oh - yes - you - will.

MRS L: *(Loudly)* Oh - no - I - will - not!

SWEENEY: *(Harshly)* You *will*. And you will do so gladly, or I shall tell that namby-pamby son of yours all about my wicked past - and yours as well! If I have read the matter aright, you have told the boy very little of our old partnership, and the way in which *you* made your reputation with pies baked from *human parts - eyes,* and *ears,* and *livers,* and other tasty bits and pieces! I shall tell him all - yes, *all*! How we robbed the customers before you cooked them!

MRS L: *(Dully)* You robbed them. *You* carved them up. *You* made me cook them. I just - sort of pretended it was ordinary meat you bought me; it was the only way I could do it... I think - I think Albert knows most of it. The gossips are not that kind.

SWEENEY: And that little girl with whom he appears to be so foolishly infatuated? Oh yes. I know all about that, I have watched them together... Shall I tell *her* about your murky past?

MRS L: It cannot be worse than my murky present. Yes - yes. All right. It seems I have no alternative. I will do your devilish work for you. My boy's happiness is at stake - and Emily's too.

SWEENEY: Why, then, me dear Mrs. L. -how very pleasant. We are partners once again. Come. Let us seal this happy bargain with a loving kiss. *(She stands like a statue, totally defeated. He lifts her lifeless hand and kisses it perfunctorily. Song, "Tango", during which he whirls her round, and she follows woodenly. Her expression one of appalled resignation.)*

SWEENEY: Dear Mrs, Lovett, you are charming;
Dear Mrs. Lovett, you're disarming;
To both of us it is alarming
That embalming is taboo.
Dear Mrs. L., you are delicious;
Dear Mrs. L., insanely vicious;
Some of my clients are suspicious,
And they wish us both adieu.
Can't you see my heart is burning?
For you and you alone it's yearning.
You are so embraceable.
Your talents irreplaceable,
I know I couldn't face a bull without you,
Dear Mrs. Lovett, why so tearful?
Dear Mrs. Lovett, let's be cheerful!
The future's bright, so don't be fearful,
'Cos I'm here, foolish and true.
So what's new?

There now! Was that not a charming little interlude? How daintily you dance, me dear - although I am quite surprised at you, singing and dancing while there is work to be done. There are two bodies in the cellar next door *(indicates door R)*, all ready for the cooking pot, and another, fresh and tender, here in this hamper. Let me show you. *(Produces a huge key from his pocket and unlocks the hamper. He lifts the lid.)* Such a pity, Ah me, so young and innocent. Not me usual type, I admit; but I could not resist the string of pearls around her pretty neck.

MRS L: *(looking in, and recoiling in horror)* I - I think I know her.

SWEENEY: *(producing a tape and expertly measuring the body)* Of course you do, my dear. You know everybody around here. Every*body*!! Ha ha!

MRS. L.:That is not very amusing, Mr. T. I think she's a friend of Miss Emily.

SWEENEY: *(carelessly)* If Miss Emily is concerned, then pray invite her to join her friend. Then she, too, will go the way of all flesh... ha ha ha! But come - you must view the contents of your new larder. *(He shuts the lid of the hamper, without locking it, then he drags a protesting Mrs. Lovett through the door R - she is moaning softly, and holding her hands over her face. Slight pause. Enter ALBERT and EMILY DL.)*

EMILY: *(as she enters, with ALBERT close behind)* I want to ask Mrs. Lovett what she thinks about it - oh! that's odd. I was certain she was down here - the girls said she was clearing up.

ALBERT: Perhaps she's in the laundry room - I'll take a look. *(He moves UL to look through door.)* No, she's not there.

EMILY: Oh well, never mind - that can wait. I'll talk to her later.

ALBERT: Emily - what *is* this all about? Why are you so excited?

EMILY:)facing him) Albert, I know who he is. I really do know who he is.

ALBERT: Who who is?

EMILY: The Ripper, of course! You *know* I have been on his trail for the past three weeks.

ALBERT: Well, yes, but...

EMILY: No, listen. You know the man calls himself Mr. Brown, the one who has taken Toby's place in your shop?

ALBERT: Yes of course I know him. And a very efficient barber he is too.

EMILY: Has it never struck you that there is something *odd* about him?

ALBERT: Odd? I don't think so. He doesn't say very much, but that's not odd, necessarily.

EMILY: Dearest - *think*!

ALBERT: Does it matter? The man is only helping out until Tobias gets back - now *there's* a mystery for you if you want one. I can't think where he's got to; it's not like him to go off like that without notice. Toby's my best friend, and he always tells me what he's doing.

EMILY: *Albert!* Mr. Brown never takes his scarf off!

ALBERT: Perhaps he feels the cold.

EMILY: *(carefully)* Is it not rumoured that Sweeney Todd bears the mark of the rope around his neck?

ALBERT: *(puzzled)* Yes?

EMILY: And he always wears a scarf to cover the mark.

ALBERT: *(staring at her as he tries to work it out)* You mean - Mr. Brown is... is Sweeney Todd?

EMILY: I am convinced of it.

ALBERT: Then Sweeney Todd - my father - has returned? After all these years! But - he is working for me! Surely he must recognise me; if it is indeed he, what has he not said anything to me?

EMILY: Because he still wanted by Scotland Yard. And Scotland Yard want the Ripper too. IF Sweeney Todd and Jack the Ripper are one and the same, it is little wonder that he is trying to conceal his identity, even from his own son.

ALBERT: *(slowly)* I suppose it is just possible that I would not have known him. I was only a child when he went away. Why did Mother say nothing to me? - oh! Perhaps that accounts for the way she has been behaving the last few days, crying, and locking herself in the laundry room. Emily - what brought you here? To this bakery, I mean? Why here particularly?

EMILY: I have had my suspicions for two days now - and I also remembered the old story about your barber's shop, and the fiendish mechanical chair which tipped the victims into the cellar below - the cellar which connected with the bakery next door. I kept watch on the shop, and in the early hours of this morning I saw him - I'm sure it was he - carrying a large bundle and sneaking into the shop. I ran across the road and looked through the window to see what he was doing, but the shop was empty!

ALBERT: There's an old stairway down to the cellar from a little room at the back.

EMILY: Aha! I thought as much! And *your* cellar adjoins *this* cellar?

ALBERT: I suppose it does. I have never really thought about it.

EMILY: Well, think of it now!

ALBERT: *(appalled)* It means my father is back to his old ways. I had hoped that, perhaps, with the passing of the years, he might have repented of his wickedness.

EMILY: *(softly)* Oh Albert - I am sorry, really I am. But the leopard will never change his spots - and if this man really is your father, you will need to be very brave in the days to come. Very brave, and very strong.

ALBERT: As long as you are here, Emily, I can face anything.

EMILY: Of course I am here - I have always known about your father, and it has never made any difference before. It will make no difference now. Albert! Look at that huge basket! What do you suppose is in there?

ALBERT: What? Where?

EMILY: A *body*, that's what! If I am right about the identity of the Ripper, then surely I must be right about this too. *(Suddenly nervous)* Go go - you open it.

ALBERT: *Me!*

EMILY: Oh, *Albert*. Oh well here goes. *(She throws back the lid and recoils in horror, with a scream. ALBERT glances in, then turns his head away. EMILY has a second look, then she and ALBERT stare at each other.)* Oh, no. No. It cannot be. It cannot. *(She has another look, then closes the lid.)* But it is! It is! In that *basket!* It is my dear friend Tilly, who disappeared on Sunday on her way to church in the fog! But why would the Ripper kill *her*? - She was a nice well brought-up girl.

ALBERT: Maybe the Ripper didn't kill her. Maybe she just died.

EMILY: In a *basket?* And - her body... mutilated? Oh, Albert - I was so excited about identifying the Ripper but this - this - *(She bursts into tears and throws* *herself into ALBERT's arms.)*

ALBERT: *(softly)* Dear Emily, don't you see? If the Ripper *is* Sweeney Todd if he is my father - then I can never ask you to marry me.*(ALBERT sings song "Be Steady". By the end, Emily has recovered her composure.)*

> Be steady now, wipe your fevered brow,
> Just consider how you can start out anew.
> Forget the pain, try to start again,
> Rainbows follow rain, and the skies will be blue.
> By sorrow you're torn, by sadness downcast,
> But tomorrow will dawn, and grief will be past.
> Remember joy, all your charms employ.
> Find another boy with a heart that is true.
> Who will love and adore,
> All the wonderful things about you.

EMILY: Albert, dear, you're very sweet, but we'll worry about all that later on, shall we? Right now, I must get down to Scotland Yard immediately, and tell them everything I know or suspect.

ALBERT: Yes, Emily. Yes, you must. But I had better come with you. If that unspeakable villain realises that you have guessed his identity, your life will be in grave danger.

EMILY: You're right. Let us all go. Mrs. Lovett, and the girls from the bakery, and we'll get Jonah and Tobias - if he has returned, of course - and anyone else we can find on the way. There is safety in numbers - we will go in a parade! *(Enter Bessie, Maisie and Lizzie DL, carrying empty trays.)* Come along, girls, we're all going on a big parade!

MAISIE: A parade!

BESSIE: Oh, goody!

LIZZIE: Where to?

EMILY: To Scotland Yard!

LIZZIE: Why there?

EMILY: To denounce Jack the Ripper - we know who he really is! *(Enter Mrs. Lovett, R; she has overheard EMILY's last remark.)*

MRS L: *(Harshly)* You are going nowhere, girls. We have a fresh batch of pies to make, and they're needed right away. *(Softening, as she sees their disappointment.)* Perhaps you can catch up with Miss Emily later, if you are quick.

EMILY: Come on, Albert - there is no time to be lost. We must go and find as many people as possible to come with us on the parade. *(They exit DL.)*

MAISIE: *(staring at the door R.)* I never knew there was a door there.

MRS L: Never you mind - it's none of your business. Get the pastry made quickly - these are *special* pies. I will get the - the *(she chokes on the word)* -the meat. *(She exits R.)*

MAISIE: There! She's gone in there again! See? Now that is odd... *(MRS. L. re-enters, carrying several red stained gauze wrapped bundles. As they work, making the pies, they sing the second part of the Pie Maker's song. MRS. L. does not join in. The girls sing wide-eyed with horror, producing bits of innards, vest, hair etc. to suit the words.)*

> Mrs. L's pies! Really the best.
> Bits of liver, pieces of vest;
> And slices of innards, all glistening red,
> Pieces of vest *(oh yes, that's wot I just said)*.
> That's wot I said, so go on and drop dead
> Sections of this! Pieces of that!
> Bits of someone's big Sunday hat!
> With small bits of gristle
> And long strands of hair,
> Left-over pieces wot shouldn't be there.
> Bits of toes and ear 'oles and eyes
> All mixed up in our luvverly pies.
> Luvverly pies! Luvverly pies!
> Ev'ry pie's a feast for your eyes.
> Such luvverly pies for you, luvverly pies!
> Be well-assured that the pastry will rise;
> Join in the fun or be cut down to size!
> Luvverly pies...luvverly pies...

(At the end, the lights dim so that the bakery is in total darkness and only the

front of the shop is lit - we are back on Fleet Street again. EMILY and ALBERT, the two policemen, the Captain, the customers, JONAH, urchins and street vendors are gathered excitedly together.)

BILL: Now then, let's make a nice orderly line, if you please sir - and you, madam.

EMILY: Is everyone here? *(She carries a banner)*

ALBERT: I'm sure the girls from the bakery will be coming as soon as they can - they wouldn't miss a parade like this! It shouldn't take them long, anyhow. Hello, Captain - I didn't see you there. Still in Town, then?

CAPTAIN: Yes, still in Town. I still have a bit of business to complete. What's all this about?

ALBERT: We'll tell you as we go.

(Enter the three street girls, L.)

FAITH: Can we join the parade?

HOPE: Have they *really* caught the Ripper?

CHARITY: Are we I time?

EMILY: Come along - everyone is welcome to join in. Let's get started. All ready? Right! Let's go!

(They all march to and fro across the front of the stage, singing "Emily's Big Crusade".)

EMILY: Now with my righteous banner
                        Lead me to the fore,
                        I'm gonna lead that big parade.
                        I know that right is right,
                        So come and join the fight -
                        It's Emily's big crusade.
                        Oh I can see it now,
                        No dragon will I fear,
                        And by no tempter I'll be swayed.
                        I know what's right and wrong,
                        My mission's mighty strong
                        For Emily's big crusade.

CHORUS:	Good old Emily, she's the one for us;
	Of no-one here is she afraid.
	She is no crank or sham,
	She doesn't care a damn.
	Join Emily's big crusade!
EMILY:	Yes, come and join me now,
	The battle must be won.
CHORUS:	She is the girl to be obeyed.
EMILY:	We've got a job to do,
	I've got a place for you
	In Emily's big parade.
CHORUS:	Good old Emily, she's our leading light,
	A shining beacon for us all.
	She won't succumb, so come and beat the drum.
	And give an answer to her call.
	Yes, we can see her now,
	No Dragon will she fear,
	And by ne tempter she'll be swayed.
	She knows what's right from wrong,
	Her mission's mighty strong,
	So join in Emily's big crusade!

(At the end of the song they all march off R, except EMILY; she stops suddenly, handing banner to last marcher.)

EMILY: I knew I'd forgotten something. I must go and have another look at poor Tilly - there was something missing . . . whatever was it? I *must* know!*(She exits front L. The lights come up again at the back, revealing the bakery; front lights dim. Enter EMILY DL.)* Ah! The basket! *(She crosses to it and lifts the lid.)* I knew it! Her pearls are missing! She always wore them - they were her grandmother's. I wondered why the Ripper would attack a well-bred girl like Tilly, but now it is clear - he murderer her for her jewels! The swine!

(Right on cue, SWEENEY enters R through hidden door. EMILY has her back to him, peering into the hamper.)

SWEENEY: Aha- ha! What have we here? *(Emily screams and leaps back.)* The meddling Miss Emily - poking your pretty little nose into things that do not concern you, eh? We'll soon put a stop to that! Perhaps you would like to join your friend - in the basket!

EMILY: You fiend! You murderer! There is blood on your hands!

SWEENEY: *(Carelessly)* Why, so there is. I must have cut myself shaving. *(Suddenly vicious;)* Into the basket!

EMILY: No! No!

SWEENEY: Yes! Yes!

EMILY: No! No! Not *that* not - not *the basket*!!

(They struggle, with mutterings of "Curse the girl!" and the like from SWEENEY, and shrieks of "No1 No!" from EMILY. Finally, EMILY swoons dramatically. NB: SWEENEY should catch her as she falls - it would be easier for him to get her into the basket than if he has to pick her up off the floor first!)

SWEENEY: Curses! The girl has swooned. Pah! There is little satisfaction in murdering an unconscious victim - I like to hear their screams of agony, and to make them feel the knife as it plunges in - ha ha ha ! He he he! More curses. Into the basket with her - I will deal with her later.

(EMILY is lowered into the basket. He shuts the lid cackling fiendishly, and exits DL. The lights dim again in the bakery, and concentrate on the front of stage - the street. The march is still in progress, the cast entering as the lights change. Reprise of "Emily's Big Crusade". ALBERT is looking worried = he goes down the line of people as they sing, searching for EMILY, and shouting above the music to make himself heard.)

ALBERT: Where's Emily? Have you seen Emily? Have *you* seen Emily? I can't find her! I can't find Emily! Emily! *Emily! (He runs off L - the parade is heading to the right point - passing the last straggler. This is a cloaked and muffled figure with a top hat. He carries a placard which says Save the Girls" As he exits R, the last of the cast to do so, and just before the curtain falls, the back of the placard comes into view - it reads "For Me!" With a nasty leer at the audience, SWEENEY exits, and the curtain falls.)*

END OF ACT II

ACT III

(Later the same day, outside the Barber's shop. The shop itself dimly lit, with no customer's; JONAH is inside, quietly tidying towels etc. It is very quiet. Hope and Charity enter DL. Looking over their shoulders and obviously scared out of their wits. Clinging together, they reach centre stage and sing the second part of their song.)

> We were once six willin' women
> Whose profession isn't slimmin',
> But now we're down to only two;
> We're no better than we should be
> And we're better than we could be,
> For there's nothing else for us to do.
> We're a brace of erring sister's
> And cater for the misters
> Who like us with our bosoms bared;
> We put up with their perversions
> And lascivious exertions -
> From humiliation we're not spared.

(Exit the two girls DR, still looming fearfully behind them. Almost immediately, the two policemen enter DR.)

BILL: hullo, they're in a hurry! Didn't even stop to pass the time of day.

FRED: They looked dead scared.

BILL: Perhaps they've seen the Ripper! *(They roar with laughter.)*

FRED: *(Sobering up suddenly)* Hey - do you think they have?

BILL: They wouldn't be walking about if they had.

FRED: There *was* only two of them. . . *(they look after the girls reflectively)* She's probably with a client.

BILL: Probably.

FRED: Have *you* found anything yet?

BILL: I haven't seen a thing. I'm not really sure I know what I'm looking for.

FRED: The Ripper, of course.

BILL: So - what does the Ripper look like?

FRED: According to the reports, he's a tall man wearing a long black cloak, a white muffler and a top hat.

BILL: But nobody seems to know what he really *looks* like, under the cloak and all that. He could be almost anybody, couldn't he? I mean, half the toffs in Town wear cloaks and top hats, and even mufflers in this foggy weather.

FRED: One report suggested he was wearing red gloves.

BILL: *Red* gloves? That's a bit unusual, ain't it?

FRED: Well, they could've been white gloves *before* he did the murders - after all, our man's never been spotted in the act, only when leaving the scene of the crimes.

BILL: Blimey. We'll need all our wits about us for this one.

FRED: *(Nudging Bill)* Promotion for the man who nabs him, eh?

BILL: And curtains for anyone who gets in his way. . . yeah great.

FRED: Here - what's this about a girl reporter from the Gazette trying to track him down?

BILL: The Raven girl? Ravin' mad if you ask me. It's true. She's always lurking about with her notebook at the ready; I've seen her down those dark alleys, not too frightened seemingly, but one of these days she'll end up as one of the Ripper's victims herself if she's not very careful.

FRED: Right. Much better to leave that sort of thing to us. Anyway, the sooner he's caught the better for all concerned. Hey - you know that young constable, Dick Smallbone? *He* thought he saw the Ripper last night and chased him down to the river.

BILL: What happened?

FRED: He fell in.

BILL: Who did - the Ripper?

FRED: Nah - the copper.

BILL: Oh well, always was a bit wet behind the ears, that one.

FRED: Wet all over he was. But that weren't all - Sergeant O'Riley was passing and went in after him to save him.

BILL: You mean Thick Mick?

FRED: Yeah, that's the one.

BILL: Go on - if it was Mick, there's bound to be more to the story.

FRED: There was. Fancies himself as a hero, doesn't he? He just dived straight in without looking and got hit by a passing barge. Ended up in hospital with a broken head.

BILL: Who fished him out?

FRED: Young Smallbone, of course. *He* didn't need rescuing - swims like a fish.

BILL: Sounds like a fishy story to me! *(They both laugh. Slight pause.)* Did you hear the rumour that Sweeney Todd's back again, *and* up to his old tricks?

FRED: Reckon Mrs. Lovett's back to baking pies for him again?

BILL: Don't - I had six this morning! Yuk. . .

FRED: *(sighing sympathetically)* A policeman's lot is not a happy one. *(They sing the Policemen's Song.)*

> We are coppers on the beat,
> Always looking for a seat;
> But we have nerves as strong as steel.
> Especially when the crook. . . shows his heels.
> We are happy in our work,
> From our duties never shirk;
> On loyalty ourselves we preen.
> We're always where the crook. . . should have been.
> We are faithful to the Law,
> 'Always hidden in a doorway.
> We are on a special task,
> For the time you mustn't ask,
> Upon this street we've often trod,
> Avoiding like the plague. . . Sweeney Todd.

There's a rumour going round
Nails and buttons have been found in
Mrs.Lovett's tasty pies,
Just imagine our surprise!
We'll do our very very best
To see if we can make. . . an arrest.

(As the song ends, Albert enters DL looking worried.)

ALBERT: Oh, thank goodness I've found you - there's *never* a policeman about when you need one. *(FRED and BILL exchange "heard -it - all - before" looks.)* I can't find Emily anywhere - that's Miss Emily Raven, she's a reporter on the Gazette, you know. She was leading our big parade to Scotland Yard to tell them about the murder, and then suddenly - well, she just wasn't there any more. What on earth do you think can have happened to her? *(While the men are talking, SWEENEY enters DR with the body of FAITH, unmistakable in her bright purple gown. Lugging bodies about is hard work, and the producer has three options here - SWEENEY can drag the girl by the hand or foot, depending upon how much she will allow! Or he can use a dummy dressed in Faith's clothes; or he can push her on in a wheelbarrow, in which case he must remember to take the wheelbarrow off-stage later. JONAH is now lolling in a chair UL reading a paper, and sees nothing. SWEENEY tiptoes carefully through the shop, and exits through the concealed door at the back, UR, with the body. Nobody sees him.)* She promised to meet me here after the parade if we got separated, but I haven't seen her since the parade started.

BILL: Oh dear.

FRED: Sounds bad.

ALBERT: She may be in danger - she has her suspicions about who the Ripper may be.

BILL: *(To Fred)* Told you, didn't I?

ALBERT: Please - you *must* help me to find her. She's such a wonderful girl, and if anything's happened to her, I - I - I don't know what I shall do.

FRED: There now , sir, don't take on so. . . She may be perfectly all right.

BILL: We'll look into it, and see what we can do.

ALBERT: There's another thing - Tobias Wragg, my assistant in the shop; he hasn't been to work for nearly three days. It's not like him at all, he's usually very reliable. And he's not at his home either. I've been there. I'm so worried about both of them - but particularly Miss Emily. *Please* do something.

FRED: We will, sir, we will. *(Aside to BILL)* Where do we start looking?

BILL: *(To FRED)* Gawd knows. . .

FRED: We'll get back to the Yard, and report these disappearances - looks like a promising lead, this does. Thank you, sir.

BILL: Cor, just when the girls are baking again - can't you smell them lovely pies? Mmmm. . .

FRED: Yeah,. But what's *in* them? That's what I'd like to know. Come on, Bill - back to the Yard.

ALBERT: You'll let me know if anything - if you find - you know?

BILL: We will keep you informed, sir.

ALBERT: Thanks. *(ALBERT exits DL, calling EMILY's name, while the policemen amble off DR. Enter SWEENEY from the concealed entrance UR. His hands are bloodied, and he is enjoying himself hugely. If a wheelbarrow has been used, he must first trundle it off DR. Then he tiptoes past JONAH and come front of stage. Centre.)*

SWEENEY: Everything is going according to me plan. Those girls of Mrs. Lovett's are busy baking- such delicious *meaty* pies! Ha ha ha! Oh, such an appetising aroma! Such a blissful bouquet! Such a phenomenal fragrance! Such a paradisial pong! And Jack the Ripper is providing the tasty ingredients. . . They're saying that the Ripper and Sweeney Todd are one and the same. Pah! Perhaps they are, perhaps they are not. Let them find out for themselves - why should I help Scotland Yard? For all they know, I *found* the bodies! Pah! I shall make it me life's work to fool them all, and to lead them a merry dance. Not just the copper's either -*all* of them! That nosy girl, the reporter; and Mrs. Lovett's puny boy. *(SWEENEY cackles happily.)* I'm leading *him* a dance all right - looking all over London for his beloved while I, Sweeney Todd, am the only one who knows where she is! They all think I am Mr. Brown the stranger, quietly at work in the shop until Tobias returns - well, they'll have a long wait. Ha ha ha! Who'll be next? Jonah, perhaps?

(SWEENEY produces a cut-throat razor and starts fingering it lovingly)
Impertinent fellow - a short- back- and -sides would become you, dear boy.
Well, perhaps not. Not yet. Me talents lie in me skill with a bright blade. . .
oh, I do enjoy being the villain! *(SWEENEY sings the Villain's Song,
punctuating it with the razor.)*

> I am a villain; wicked as hell.
> Ready and willin' bodies to sell.
> Parting the top of your head -
> I do it well,
> I am a devil, sharp as they come;
> Barber of Seville? Figure of fun!
> You want to die in your bed?
> I'll get it done.
> Here comes a victim, ready to pluck;
> I'll try to constrict 'im; I fancy me luck.
> I am a fleecer after his cash.
> What'll it be, sir? Short back and bash?
> By ugly tales you're misled,
> Go on - be rash!
> My reputation couldn't be worse,
> No hesitation into the hearse.
> I am a twister riddled with vice.
> Slaughter me sister? Wouldn't think twice.
> Everywhere smothered in red -
> Isn't it nice? So nice!

*(At the end of the song, SWEENEY folds the razor and puts it in his pocket
as he turns to go. He almost bumps into MRS.LOVETT who has entered DL.)*

SWEENEY: Ah- haa! Whom have we here? *(Strokes moustache)* None other
than me old friend and partner, eh, Mrs.L.?

MRS L: *(pushing him away)* I've had enough of this, Sweeney Todd. That poor
girl! I'd know that purple dress anywhere. How *could* you?

SWEENEY: *(Dangerously polite)*Me dear Mrs. Lovett - how could I *what*? You
think I would demean meself, to use me talents on a common woman of the
streets?

MRS L: You brought her in here, there's no denying that. All bloody, and. . . oh, oh, oh. . . *(She dissolves into tears.)*

SWEENEY: You think to sway me with your crocodile tears, woman? Come, Mrs.L.,you never used to be so fastidious. And your pies have never smelled so delicious - so utterly glorious, so ambrosial, so celestial!

MRS L: Flattery will get you nowhere, Sweeney. I mean it - I just can't take any more, even if it means I must go to gaol again. I'm going to Scotland Yard. *(She tries to push pat him.)*

SWEENEY: Oh no you are not, me fine friend. *(He grabs her arm and brandishing the razor at her.)* Unless you wish to find yourself baked into one of your own tasty pies - because I shall have no mercy on any who seek to betray me. Believe me, me dear Mrs. L., believe me. . .

MRS L: *(defeated)* I believe you.

SWEENEY: Back to your kitchen then, and continue the work for which I pay you.

MRS L: Pay me? *Pay* me? When have I ever seen the colour of your money? Not that I would take your dirty money anyway, not now, not when it's earned in blood.

SWEENEY: *(casually)* Wasn't it always? Fie, Mrs. L., I swear you are becoming quite melodramatic. Let us have no more of it - to your kitchen! *(She exits DL, sobbing.)* Curses! Damnation to the woman! How dare she bandy arguments with *me*? I'll make her bake her pies till the crack of doom! *(Exit SWEENEY DR, cursing and cackling horribly. Pause. Enter Charity, scared stiff, DR. She sings the final verse of the Street Girls Song.)*

CHARITY:

I'm a solitary floosie
And although I'm not so choosy
I'm very careful who I see;
If the Ripper comes here looking
For a cemetery booking -
I shall buzz off like the proverbial bee.
Yes, I'm going - just in case it's me!

(Exits DL. The girl scuttles off. Enter the two policemen, DR, as the lights come up a little in the shop area.)

BILL: Mr. Todd - Albert! Are you there?

JONAH: *(Looking up)* You looking for Albert?

BILL: Yes - is he around?

JONAH: Nah. *(Retreats behind his newspaper again.)*

FRED: Do you know where we can find him?

JONAH: *(without moving)* Nah.

FRED: *(mildly sarcastic)* Thanks for your help. Ah, *there* you are, sir *(to ALBERT as he enters DL.)* We was just looking for you.

ALBERT: Have you found her? Have you found Emily? I'm sure she's not far away - I can *feel* it. . . in fact, I thought I heard her calling just now, but I still can't find her. Jonah, have *you* seen Emily?

JONAH: Huh?

ALBERT: *(Impatiently)* Emily: have you *seen* her?

JONAH: Nah.

ALBERT: Oh for heaven's sake, Jonah, put down that scandal sheet and come and help me to look for her. Oh! *(To the policemen)* Did you want me for something? *(Jonah gets up reluctantly and ambles forward to stage centre, front, with ALBERT, FRED and BILL. During the ensuing dialogue, and unseen by the others, SWEENEY lugs on stage the body of HOPE in her bright yellow dress, and deposits her through the concealed door at the back of the shop. He then lurks in the shadows just inside the open shop front, overhearing the conversation having first pushed barrow off-stage, if one has been used.)*

BILL: Just to tel you we haven't come across any clues yet, but we've reported the missing person to the Yard.

FRED: *(importantly)* We're officially on the case now.

JONAH: What's all the fuss about?

ALBERT: Emily's disappeared and we can't find her anywhere.

JONAH: That's odd. . .

ALBERT: Odd? What is? Have you thought of something?

JONAH: Yes.

ALBERT: What *is* it then? Do you know where she is?

JONAH: Nah.

ALBERT: *Jonah!!* What *is* it that's odd?

JONAH: Well, it makes *two,* don't you see? *(He intercepts ALBERT's furious look and hurries on.)* *Two* wot have disappeared, like. Vanished. Miss Emily and Tobias.

BILL: *(To FRED)* Thought he had something there, didn't you?

FRED: For a minute, I did.

ALBERT: Lord, yes, I'm worried about Tobias, of course I am, he's my best friend; but he can take care of himself, Emily's just a girl, and she's found out about the Ripper and I'm so afraid he might have caught her, and done something to her to silence her.

JONAH: Oh. Yeah. You're right to be worried. They say the Ripper likes carving up girls.

ALBERT: *(bitterly)* Oh, you *are* a Job's comforter. Thank you very much.

JONAH: Actually, I think I did hear something a little while back.

ALBERT: You did? What did you hear?

JONAH: Well, like somebody calling for help. I think.

ALBERT: What did it sound like?

JONAH: *(In a faint falsetto voice)* Help, help.

ALBERT: It must be she! It must be! Where did the voice come from? Jonah - could it have been Emily's voice?

JONAH: Well. . .

BILL: Speak up, man, this is important.

ALBERT: Of *course* it's important - think, Jonah, think!

JONAH: Ummm. . . *(While he is thinking about it, the others are listening with baited breath for his answer, a faint cry for help is heard.)* Like that! Just like that!

ALBERT: That was Emily's voice - I'm certain of it! But where *is* she? Oh! *(He claps his hand to his face)* I wonder. . .

FRED: *(Really on the ball)* You've thought of something, sir?

ALBERT: I'm thinking about that ghastly basket in my mother's kitchen - the one with the body in it.

BILL: Body? Why Body?

FRED: First we've heard of a body in Mrs. L's kitchen. Pies, yes; bodies, no.

BILL: Unless. . .

FRED: *(Cottoning on)* - unless Mrs. L's at it again, and Sweeney Todd really has come back!

BILL: Did you recognise the body, sir?

ALBERT: Yes. A young girl, a friend of Emily's, Tilly, I think she was called.

BILL: That might be Miss Matilda Mordiford, her what's been reported missing from home by her Ma.

FRED: A *dead* body, was it, sir?

ALBERT: *(shuddering)* Oh yes. With the mark of the Ripper upon it - unmistakably.

BILL: You didn't think to mention this before, sir?

ALBERT: We were on our way to Scotland Yard to tell you when Emily vanished and I was so worried about *her* that I forgot all about the - the other.

BILL: Hmmm. *(Another faint cry is heard.)*

ALBERT: There it is again! It sounds as though it's coming from the pie-shop kitchen - follow me! *(He runs off DL, followed by the policemen drawing their truncheons).*

JONAH: *(alone and suddenly feeling nervous)* Oo-er. *(He follows the others at the double. SWEENEY comes to the front of stage, centre, trying to wipe the blood from his hands.)*

SWEENEY: Curses! They'll find the girl - and the body of her friend! But the girl lives - they can't accuse me of murdering *her*! No, but they'll accuse me of all the Ripper's crimes if they catch me, and they will send me to the gallows and make sure I do not escape the rope a second time. Curses! And more curses!

(Enter Captain Thumbtickle, DL.)

CAPTAIN: *(breathlessly)* Who's that? Oh Mr Brown, it's just you - you gave me quite a start, standing there like that. They say there's been another murder, another one of those poor street girls.

SWEENEY: *(brightening)* Oh yes? Where?

CAPTAIN: In Whitechapel, like the rest. Just outside the 'Dog and Duck'.

SWEENEY: Ah-hah!

CAPTAIN: Where is everybody? I thought I might find young Albert here.

SWEENEY: Albert is . . . is below.

CAPTAIN: Below?

SWEENEY: *(gesturing with his thumb)* Below.

CAPTAIN: Has he found Miss Emily yet? He was in quite a state when I saw him half an hour ago.

SWEENEY: Yes, I believe he has found her.

CAPTAIN: Oh, I'm glad.

SWEENEY: Yes.

(The conversation flags. The CAPTAIN finds SWEENEY's stillness puzzling, and SWEENEY is pondering on his own problems. There is a sudden commotion as ALBERT bursts onto the stage DL, half carrying a dishevelled EMILY in his arms. He is followed by the policemen - carrying the hamper, which they set down on stage - JONAH, MRS LOVETT, and her three pie girls.)

ALBERT: I've found her! I've found Emily! Oh Emily, I'm so glad you're all right - I was desperately afraid for you. Look, Mr Brown, I've found her! Loom, Captain!

BILL: We've got half of Scotland Yard out looking for you, young lady.

JONAH: Which half?

("Mr Brown" turns away and slides back into the shadowy doorway of the shop.)

CAPTAIN: There, she's looking better already.

ALBERT: Emily, Emily darling, are you all right? Can you hear me? Speak to me!

EMILY: Of course I can hear you, Albert. I should think the whole of Fleet Street can hear you. Don't make such a fuss. Oh, just *look* at the state of my skirt! It's all covered in dust, and all those red stains -oh! It must be blood. . . poor dear Tilly. Oh Albert, it really was rather horrid being locked into that dreadful basket with a dead body!

JONAH: *(helpfully)* At least it was someone you knew.

ALBERT: *Jonah*! Be Quiet!

JONAH: *(Amiably)* All right.

EMILY: Have they caught him yet? Did the parade get to Scotland Yard?

CAPTAIN: There's just been another murder reported.

EMILY: Then the *haven't* caught him yet. The fiend! The foul, devilish, murdering fiend!

LIZZIE: *Another* murder?

MAISIE: Another *murder?*

BESSIE: I wonder who it was this time? I hope it wasn't someone we know.

MRS L: That's enough, girls. Go and see if you can help Miss Emily. *(The girls help EMILY to dust herself down and straighten her clothing.)*

EMILY: Thank you - thank you.

MRS L: *(raising her voice)* Come out, Sweeney Todd; come out and face the music. Don't think we can't see you, skulking in that doorway. We know you're there.

SWEENEY: *(Stepping forward)* Do you mean me, Madam? I am Mr. Brown the barber, and I have never seen you before in me life.

MRS L: A barber maybe, but Sweeney Todd nonetheless. And *(Bitterly)* who should know better than I? *(Every one murmurs in amazement- except*

EMILY.)

EMILY: Ah-hah! I *thought* so! *(The policemen close in on SWEENEY.)*

ALBERT: So *you* are Sweeney Todd? My - my father?

MRS L: *(Stridently) Never* your father, boy.

ALBERT: Never - but - what do you mean? *Not* my father?

MRS L: Certainly not. My relationship with Mr. Todd has always been a strictly business one.

ALBERT: Then -if *he's* not my father, who is?

MRS L: It's a long story - perhaps later. . .

ALBERT: No! I have waited too long already? Tell me now.

MRS L: Very well. After my first husband died, Mr. Lovett as was, I met a man called Nelson Thumbtickle. He was not much to look at *(The CAPTAIN reacts indignantly)* But he was kind and generous so I married him. One day I sent him out to the King's Head for a quart of ale - and he never came back. Eventually I fetched the ale myself, and changed my name back to Lovett as I didn't much fancy being called Mrs. Thumbtickle. Then I opened this pie shop, with Sweeney Todd the barber next door. When Albert was born soon afterwards, everyone assumed the child was Sweeney's - and somehow it seemed easier to let them think so. I didn't know then what an evil, black-hearted monster he was to become.

ALBERT: My name is - Albert *Thumbtickle?*

MRS L: Albert Horatio Thumbtickle.

ALBERT: And Sweeney Todd is *not* my father? I do *not* bear his tainted blood?

MRS L: Not one sticky drop.

ALBERT: Emily, oh Emily! Do you hear that? I *can* ask you to marry me after all! If you'll have me; could you bear to become Mrs. Thumbtickle? *Will* you marry me?

EMILY: Darling Albert, of course I will. You can always change your name later.

(She and ALBERT sing a duet, a reprise of "The Boy/Girl I Love".)

EMILY	ALBERT	
Canto Fermo	Alternative A	Alternative B
	In my loving arms You'll always be In the warmth of my caress.	In my loving arms You'll always be In the warmth of my caress.
Now your loving heart belongs to me we shall find true happiness		
For you my love know what my feelings are.	Now that you are mine and in love with me, see what my feelings are for you.	And you my love know why I feel as bright as any star in skies above.
And now I've found The answer to my cry.	Now I've found the answer to my cry, a cry to God above,	You are the answer to my prayer. You are the object of my fervent love.
It's you my love, I keep dreaming of	You alone I love my love. It's You I'm always dreaming of,	Yes, you, my love, will be my dream of heaven above.
For I know you will provide me with the love that's been denied me, and you'll stay right here beside me till I die.	Because I'm sure you will provide me with the love that has been denied me, and you'll stay right here beside me till I die.	And now I'm sure you will provide me with the love that has been denied me, and you'll stay right here beside me till I die.

CAPTAIN: *(stepping forward)* I am delighted to see these two young people so happily betrothed. And Mrs. Lovett - dear Mrs.Lovett - has resolved the puzzle I have been engaged in trying to unravel over these past few days. *(To her)*Do you not recognise me, my dear?

MRS L: Recognise you? No, wait! Can it be? No. Is it? No. Yes! It is! It is! Nelly! My own dear Nelly Thumbtickle back from the dead!

CAPTAIN: Not dead, my dear, just press-ganged. . .

JONAH: From Fleet street!

CAPTAIN: I sailed the seven seas, did passing well for myself and now own my own ship. Captain Nelson Thumbtickle at your service, my dear wife.

MRS L: Land sakes! Nelly! I can't believe it! After twenty years! Where's that quart of ale I sent you out for? My, but you've changed so much. . . is it really you?

CAPTAIN: *(smiling)* The proof is where it always was. Do you not remember that we Thumbtickles all bear a birthmark on our - well, in a peculiar place?

MRS L: *(blushing)* Oh! Yes, how could I forget. . . and Albert has one in exactly the same place.

ALBERT: *(blushing too)* Oh, Ma!

EMILY: *(to Albert)* Where? Show me!

ALBERT: *(without taking his eyes off the Captain)* On our wedding night, dearest.

EMILY: Oooooh. . .

ALBERT: Father? Father!

CAPTAIN: My son! At last! *(They embrace.)*

ALBERT: And now for Sweeney Todd, whose very existence has made my life a misery. All my life I have been branded as the son of a murderer: Mother, how could you let me go through all that?

MRS L: I thought it was for the best. Nelly had vanished and I thought he must be dead. It is not easy for a woman to bring up her child alone. Sweeney was there, in the shop next door, and to give the scoundrel his due he was kind enough to me in those early days before he started blackmailing me into making his nauseating pies.

ALBERT: *(to Sweeney)* And you! You let me think it too!

SWEENEY: *(with an unrepentant sneer)* Having a brat around added a nice touch of respectability to *me* background.

JONAH: Not all that respectable, when we all knew you was never married. *(SWEENEY glares at him and lunges towards him. The policemen try to stop him, and in the tussle BILL dislodges SWEENEY's scarf.)*

EMILY: *(Pointing dramatically)* Look! Look! The mark of the rope! There is no doubt whatsoever that you are that notorious villain, Sweeney Todd!

SWEENEY: Curse the girl! All right - I admit it. I *am* Sweeney Todd. But not this bloody murderer, this Jack the Ripper. You have nothing on me! Sweeney Todd was hanged, remember? Hanged! And there's the scar to prove it. You cannot hang a man twice!

FRED: *(to BILL)* Can't you?

BILL: If we can't, it won't be for want of trying. *(Clamping his hand on SWEENEY's shoulder)* I arrest you inn the name of the Law.

SWEENEY: *(Throwing him aside)* Not before I have taken me revenge on the cause of all me misfortunes! *(He brandishes a knife and stabs MRS LOVETT, who screams and staggers back.)* Take that! And that! And that! Die, you harridan, die!

(All the men leap forward to restrain him, except ALBERT who kneels by his mother, now prostrate on the ground.)

ALBERT: Mother! Mother! Speak to me! Please, please do not die!

CAPTAIN: *(Joining ALBERT)* After all these years, when we are so newly united, do not leave us, dearest wife!

MRS L: *(painfully)* It takes more than a murderous swine like Sweeney Todd to kill *me*! I'll live - if it's only to make sure he swings!

SWEENEY: Curses! Let me get at her!

MRS L: I can tell you now what happened. . .

ALBERT: Happened? What happened?

MRS L: To Tobias. . .

SWEENEY: Hold your tongue, you garrulous hag!

MRS L: He was murdered - murdered. . .*(she falls back.)*

SWEENEY: *(pleased)* Hah!

ALBERT; Oh, Mother!

BILL: Yes, yes? Who by?

FRED: Who murdered Tobias?

MRS L: *(Reviving)* I saw it happen - I saw it all. . .

ALL: Yes, yes? *(She falls back. All groan. She revives.)*

MRS L: I saw him kill Tobias. . . poor Tobias. . .

SWEENEY: Blast!

ALL: Yes yes?

MRS L: All that blood. . . *(her mind is wandering)*

BILL: *Who?* Who killed Tobias?

MRS L: It was - he! Sweeney Todd! Sweeney Todd murdered poor Tobias. There! Now I can die happy.

SWEENEY: Curses. And more curses.

JONAH: Mrs. L. Will be the death of you, Sweeney.

(SWEENEY snarls at him, cursing. ALBERT, EMILY and the CAPTAIN are tending to MRS.L., who looks fairly healthy under the circumstances; ALBERT stands up and faces SWEENEY.)

ALBERT: You dirty dog! Tobias was my best friend.

JONAH: Mine too.

ALBERT: You devil! You monstrous, Machiavellian murderer! You fiend incarnate!

JONAH: You filthy beast! You swine!

BILL: *(To FRED.)* I still reckon he's the Ripper, don't you?

FRED: I reckon. The judge will decide. Got him fair and square for Tobias anyway - just so long's the old lady don't snuff it. Got the knife?

BILL: The knife? Yes. Nice bit of evidence, that.

SWEENEY: *(with despairing hand-to brow gesture.)* Oh God, the basket. What may still be in the basket? Ahem! *(To all, carelessly)* Are the *diamonds* still at the bottom of the *basket? (All stare at him.)*

BILL: What diamonds?

SWEENEY: *(Thinking quickly)* Um - der - a *wonderful* diamond necklace, worth a kings ransom. . . *(The policemen make a dive at the basket, throw open the lid - everyone reacts to the 'smell' - and starts searching. The odd arm or leg may be thrown out, with appropriate reactions from the cast.)*

You seem to be somewhat - er- *hampered* by your cloak and helmet; do allow me to hold them for you. *(He crosses to the basket as he speaks. FRED hands him his cloak and helmet.)* Permit me also to relieve you of your *truncheon! (SWEENEY grabs FRED's truncheon, and briskly bops both coppers on the head with it. Then he shoves them so that they both fall head-first into the basket - he drops the lid on them, slaps the helmet on his own head, his top hat falling off. A bit of business could be included here, with one of the girls picking it up and putting it on the another's head. SWEENEY heads for the exit DL, shouting;)* You'll never catch me now! Ha ha ha! He he he! *(He exits at the run.)*

BILL: *(Struggling from the basket)* After him! Quick!

  FRED: *(Getting tangled up with BILL)* Don't let him get away! *(Everyone, with the exception of MRS.LOVETT, joins in the chase. They all hare off after SWEENEY, leaping lightly over MRS.L's prostrate body. Ast one point she tries to sit up, only to be flattened in the rush. The mechanics of the chase will depend on the stage facilities and the ingenuity of the producer. SWEENEY is always slightly ahead, chuckling evilly, and yelling "Catch me if you can!" Finally, everyone ends up on stage - except SWEENEY.)*

BILL: We've lost him!

FRED: There goes our promotion.

BILL: Don't worry, we'll get him. He can't get far.

EMILY: I don't care about Sweeney Todd *or* Jack the Ripper any more, now that I've got Albert!

ALBERT: Emily - darling! *(They fall into each other's arms. Blackout. Green spotlight, DR, on SWEENEY, who is still wearing the policeman's clothes.)*

SWEENEY: *(Gleefully)* I've *foiled* 'em again! Ha ha ha! He he he! They will *never know* if I am Jack the Ripper - or *not!* Ha ha ha! He he he! *(Maniacal cackling as the spotlight fades. Blackout. Then a harsh white spotlight blazes on the stage, this time DL, on a complete stranger wearing black cloak, top hat, etc, and lovingly caressing a huge gleaming knife.)*

MAN: *(In a deep, deliberate voice) Is* Sweeney Todd Jack the Ripper? Or could it be - *someone else?*

(Blackout., After a moment, the lights gradually come up again as the opening bars of the final chorus are played. All the cast (with the exception of SWEENEY and the MAN) come on and take their places; the street vendors, customers and other 'extras' in the back row, with FAITH, HOPE and CHARITY, BILL and FRED, MAISIE, BESSIE and LIZZIE. JONAH and TOBIAS, in the next row. In the front row are the CAPTAIN and MRS. LOVETT, and ALBERT and EMILY - with a space between them for SWEENEY, whose final entrance should be as dramatic as possible. The final chorus is sung by all.)*

> Goodbye Sweeney, the peelers are after you;
> Scarper away 'cos the beadle's about,
> Farewell Sweeney, the end is in sight;
> It's time to be off without a doubt.
> 'Bye Mrs. Lovett, just keep up your laughter do;
> Coping with Sweeney you've been a good scout.
> Ciao Mrs. Lovett, you fought a good fight;
> It's time to be off without a doubt.
> Your time is running out fast,
> The Law is making a stand.
> And the justice will triumph at last
> When you two are taken in hand.
> Au'voir, Ripper, your doings ain't half taboo;
> How many strumpets have gone up the spout?
> Ripper? Sweeney? I've just seen the light.
> There's plenty to learn about. . . be off!
> And show concern about. . . be off!
> We'd best do a turnabout somehow. . . be off and how!
> It's time to be off and out now. . . be off!
> Right now!. . . be off now!

THE CURTAIN FALLS

PRODUCTION NOTES

Production notes are, of course, mainly to assist the inexperienced producer; however, even the experts may find them helpful in some respects. Victorian melodrama, especially this 'tongue-in-cheek' variety, is a wonderful opportunity for the actors to ham it up; the producer must not let them go over the top - every actor must believe totally in the part he or she is playing, and act with the greatest sincerity, albeit rather over-dramatising. The audience must be encouraged to hiss and boo the villain and cheer the hero and heroine. The villain is expected to hiss back at the audience. It's not a bad idea to plant friends in the audience to lead the barracking, or even to cast somebody as a 'stagehand' to come on with a board saying "Hiss", "Boo", or "cheer" whenever a reaction is required. Stage directions have been given throughout the script, merely as a guide to producers in a well-equipped theatre, and the other more appropriate for the village hall performance. On a fair-sized stage, one set will suffice for the entire play, so long as there is room for the Barber Shop and the Pie Shop to be placed side by side, with lighting indicating where the action is taking place. On a small stage, Acts 1 and 3 will include the Barber Shop, and ACT II the Pie Shop. *(See illustrations)* We have seen this play performed with a cast of sixty, which was very effective in the crowd scenes, but the minimum number should be about 30, with 16 speaking parts *(8 Male, 8 Female)* Tobias can double The Stranger, if he is tall enough. At the end, the audience should think that The Stranger is Sweeney - until he turns round and speaks; the question they should then be asking themselves is - is this Jack the Ripper? Sweeney should be a tall and menacing figure, with a large moustache to twirl. Mrs Lovett should be plumpish *(all those pies)*, and Emily a 'modern miss' - but she must remember she is a Victorian miss. The three pie girls should be vivacious and flirtatious *(with the two policemen, who are rather cowardly and not very bright)* The three street girls can be as saucy as they like, in low cut gowns in purple, scarlet and yellow. *(This is important to the action of the play, as they should be instantly recognisable by the colour of their dresses. Most lighting effects are suggested in the body of the script, but if a village hall really cannot rise to anything more complicated than the odd spotlight, the right effects can be achieved by some characters 'freezing' while the others are acting in a separate scene which would normally be indicated by lighting. A green spotlight on the villain is always a plus! If the two cubicle "shops" are used on a single set, then they should be lit separately, in accordance with which one is the centre of action at the time. If there are no front tabs, blackouts may be used to indicate the end of the acts. A Victorian London backdrop would be ideal, but then play can just as easily be done in curtains or whatever the producer can devise. So much depends on the facilities of the hall or theatre available, and on the ingenuity of the set designer. Full stage lighting for the street scenes, except Act 1 scene 2, which is "evening"; a mock-up of a Victorian street gaslight would be great, if possible! Furniture is basic - three chairs in the Barber Shop, and a table for jugs and basins, towels, combs, and cut-throat razors (for safety reasons, these need not be the real thing, cardboard cut-outs will do!)* In the Pie Shop, a counter or table must be provided, with a mock-up of a large black leaded range at the back., and a large skip or hamper at the side,, bearing a huge padlock. The opening chorus should include the entire cast except Sweeney; the pie girls can be selling their pies, the policeman arresting pickpockets, etc.

PROPERTIES

ACT I

Opening chorus: It will depend on the producer and/or the musical director as to which street vendors are included in the scene; if the nine are cast, the props needed will be:-

A trug-like basket for the lavender seller

A Victorian knife-grinding "machine"

Cloth-covered baskets for the pie girls

A cloth-covered basket for the "eels"

A neck-tray for the match seller

A workman's apron and hammer/chisel for the hair mender

A trug for the other flower seller

Basket of oranges/lemons for the fruit seller

The Town Crier should have a hand bell

Emily needs a school exercise book and pencil *(spiral-bound note-books were not used in the 1890's)*

The barber's shop: Three chairs, towels, bowls, comb and scissors, mirror, a newspaper "The Whitechapel Gazette"

Sweeney has a blood-stained dagger

Signs for Stagehand if needed, i.e "Later that evening"

ACT II

A trestle table or two, depending on the size of the stage

"ovens", either painted or mock-up's - ideally these should have an opening door and shelves for the pies, but with a simple set the pie girl can hide most of the business by turning her back on the audience, and "taking out" the same tray which she has just put in to a painted oven. Her acting should indicate which tray is hot and which tray is cold!

Rolling pins, mixing bowls and wooden spoons, large jars marked 'flour', 'sugar', 'salt', dripping (these too can be mock-up's, real, or painted on the backdrop)

Some real flour and pieces of dough should ne used if possible in the slapstick scene

A few real jam tarts and meat pies *(small)* for the policemen man to eat

A large skip or hamper, with a huge padlock

A bucket *(not plastic)*

Enormous key for Sweeney to open "padlock"

Tape measure for Sweeney

For Mrs Lovett - one or two blood-stained packages *(wrapped in old sheets or similar)*

The girls can mime the 'hairs' and smaller and unpleasant contents of the pies, but 'bits of vest' and something 'glistening red' should be provided

For Emily - a banner or placard on a pole saying "Votes for Women"

For Sweeney - placard on a pole : "Save the girls" on one side and "for me!" on the other

ACT II

Sweeney needs a life size rag doll dressed in purple to match Faith's gown *(a rough approximation will do)*

A wheelbarrow if the producer decides to use one

A cut throat razor

Jonah needs a newspaper again

Sweeney - a rag doll, this time in yellow to match Hope's dress

Wheelbarrow if wanted

Policemen carry on the hamper, containing an arm and a leg

Sweeney - a knife or dagger, the plastic sort where the blade disappears into the handle when used to stab is probably the safest

A large gleaming knife or chopper for the Stranger

COSTUMES

Generally speaking, all the characters should be dressed in the style of the late 19th Century, but if finances are short - and they usually are - an approximation of the period will give the right effect. For the women long full skirts, some perhaps with a bustle behind; high necked, long sleeved blouses; bonnets would also have to worn outdoors, but a certain amount of licence can be taken with this - the shop girls and the street girls can do without hats, so can Mrs Lovett. Emily could have a straw hat hanging down her back from ribbons tied beneath her chin *(she'll have to lose the hat when she goes into the hamper!)* A cameo brooch at her throat would be suitable. Most women wore high buttoned boots in those days, but they would certainly be hard to come by today. Some of the daintier ankle length styles of heeled ladies boots might suffice *(nobody will notice the zip in place of tidy buttons)* otherwise a simple slipper *(like a ballet shoe)* or court shoe might be best. Platform soles , bovver boots and trainers are definitely out. Mrs Lovett should wear a large white apron over her skirt and the pie girls, who should be modestly dressed in colours which cannot be mistaken for those of the street girls, should also have aprons. The three street girls wear low cut satiny dresses in bright colours - Faith purple, Hope, yellow, and Charity scarlet. The dresses can be as sexy as the period would allow, and Hope should wear a garter to be displayed while flirting with the policemen. The street vendors would probably have sacking aprons over their skirts. The men would mostly wear breaches and boots, with a collarless shirt, waistcoat and cap; perhaps a neckerchief. This would be suitable for Albert, Jonah and Tobias. Sweeney must wear a top hat and full evening dress, with a long black cloak; white evening scarf *(Muffler)* and blood-stained white gloves. His make-up must include a vivid red scar around his throat, and a large moustache to twirl. His features should be rather pale, with dark eyebrows. The Stranger should be dressed identically to Sweeney, but his make-up should not include a scar or moustache - a small neat beard could be worn. Captain Thumbtickle's costume should be vaguely nautical, breaches, jacket etc; and he should wear a hat *(which he would of course remove in the presence of ladies)* He might carry a silver topped cane, or even a telescope if he wishes. The policemen wear the uniforms of the period with the tall hats, and carry truncheons on their belts. If in doubt about period costume, the local reference library will always be able to provide books on the subjects so that they may be as authentic as possible.